Nieren-Diät-Kochbuch für Anfänger:

365 Tage einfache und schmackhafte Rezepte für eine natrium-, kalium- und phosphorarme Diät zur Bewältigung von Nierenerkrankungen

Rhea Rosenweg

"For those pesky FBI agents trying to incite violence with their fake accounts. On social media platforms worldwide trying take our rights away, make sure you're not ill informed this way."

The storm is almost here...

Trump 2024...In November he will win again...the end.

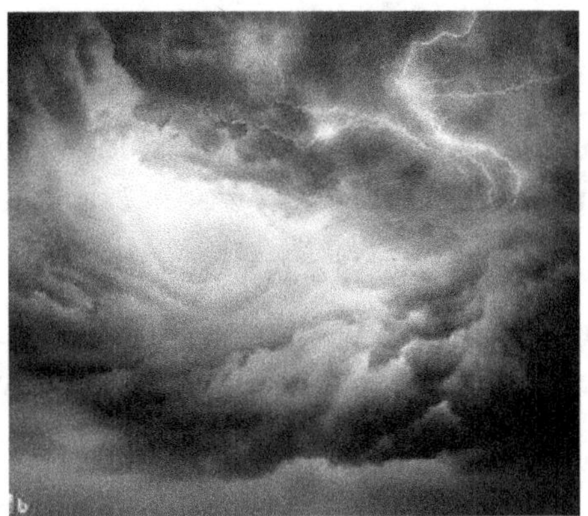

Political Madness is coming in July 2024.

MAGA (the untold story of Trump and his supporters). Coming in November 2024.

Join me on YouTube and Rumble...

Added Note:

Poetry allows our struggles, sorrows, sadness, happiness, love, inspiration, to flood the pages of poetry. We instill those emotions and feelings into words...so many people around the world can relate too.

I have always enjoyed writing poems in my spare time...now you get to see the inside of my head...how I see the reality of living life in this awesome world.

Politics are driven into our living rooms, office buildings, radio stations, or wherever you are during the day...

One side seems to hate America, our foundational principles, and wants to reform this country into a Democracy.

The other side of the Political spectrum, sees our struggles, gives us false hope online, but nothing seems to ever help the ongoing reality we all live in... Politicians on both sides of the spectrum seem to be as one unit...undermining our realization of how we live, and what situations we survive under.

Whatever side you vote for, or whoever you support or dislike. One thing is for sure...Your taxes will be well spent...long before they even collect them. We are trillions in debt, and those who handle our taxes have a spending problem. When that gets under control...our way of life will improve...until then...keep reading these Political poems, posting on social media, and spreading the word about America and our Constitutional Republic. How we need real leadership to make America Great Again.

Have a wonderful day/night wherever you are in the world...coffee drinkers.

Signing off...until tomorrow.

Bonus Poem...

The Storm

"Trump will wreak havoc on those who are corrupt. Fire everyone involved in the deep state's cover up. America will finally be first again."

"That day will be so grand...time to finally make a united stand. Against those who seek to destroy this wonderful land. At the voting booth...silly undercover decoys...trying to play their liberal hands."

Watch out...

Thank you to my wonderful wife...you are a godsend. I love you deeply.

Thank you to my social media family...you mean more to me than you know...Thank you all for being a part of this journey as well.

Thank you to Amazon for allowing me to reach the world with my writings.

Thank you to all the men/women in the military/police. Without your sacrifice, this country would not have lasted this long.

We owe everything to you all...God Bless.

Finally...

Thank you to everyone in the world, who has purchased my novels in the past, and who supports my writing career in the present/future. Without you, I wouldn't be able to reach the world. In all 127 countries in the world, who have either read/purchased my novels/poetry. You are all honored...Thank you...coffee drinkers.

Next Series Book

(25 + 1 Poems) Inspirational Book of Christian Poems.

Look for this book out around June 2024.

Finding Jesus will be out in March 2024.

"Liberals have ruined their own last 8 years, drinking from a murky sewage water foundation, banking on a Trump conviction. Everything, even the kitchen sink was thrown, nothing can stop MAGA...keep that Blown Witch Hunt coming."

"Fake Impeachments, Endless investigations, Liberals are cowards, hellbent on control. Trying to break this country's will by dividing this nation. Even if a social collapse happens, they do not care. They are right, you are wrong, their Democracy will live on."

"Trump was right about near everything. WWIII, open borders, even an economic disaster. Just to name a few...that you won't hear on your biased evening news."

"Fake fact-checkers, judges, and lawyers united. In the biggest Election Interference this world has ever seen. Too bad Trump will still win in the end. Because the People elect who we want to represent. Not a few Politicians at Biden's Late-night Pizza party basement buffet."

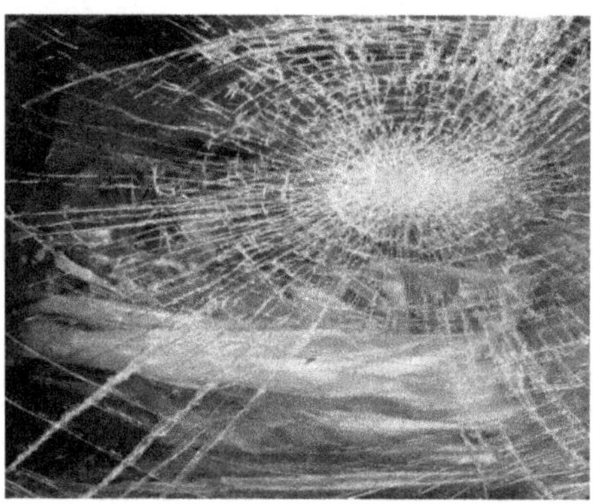

Thank You...

Thanks for being here on this journey of writing these political poems. This will include the first series of poems. I will begin writing the next (25 poems) series soon after publishing.

There will be (4) sets of poems totaling 100 in all. Each poem will be written by my hands/mind. I used no AI during the writing of these poems.

By the time this book gets released, I will have welcomed my 11,000th follower on X formally known as Twitter. I really enjoy writing poetry, as it brings comfort to my mind, in this ever-chaotic world we live in now.

Thank you to my family and friends, who all support my journey to becoming a professional in my field of writing.

"Reasoning behind this poem"

Every state in these United States has a right to protect its citizens...Texas is no different. This poem was written in support of a state's right to defend its own people who reside there. I hope Texas continues to defend its people. As it should...always."

24. Taxpayer

"Electric, gas, water, rent, even toilet paper...shit money goes fast. Taxed forever by those who shred our dollars, endless spending, driven by greed, understanding their need. To milk our funds before they are collected. On wars, illegals, other country's social delinquents."

"Americans are banks to those who seed. Foundations marked for profit. Preventing us from moving forward. We are a nation built for slaves, sinking under our own bottomless pit. Of desperation and despair...Outcast from society, until next February."

"America only takes the best. Unless you have too much debt. We'll take your home, vehicles, and land. Let us talk when you have the time. Please just sign on this dotted line."

"Yard Sales, Fleamarket, Tips and more. Taxes for every lost soul. Government has complete and total control."

"Congrats...Taxpayer you are welcomed with wide open arms. Spend more, pay more, even after you are gone. Give me that Dollar...here is your 20 cents back. No need to thank me...We are from the IRS."

"Reasoning behind this Poem"

"I wrote this poem in honor of all the taxpayers...who suffer from the economic disaster of this administration's spending problem. Everything, from the cost of food to gas has gone up. When in your lifetime, has it been this terrible to be able to support your families. I've had to stand in long food lines, waiting to be fed. Because the cost of food in grocery stores nationwide is just too unaffordable."

Thanks...coffee drinkers.

25. Witch Hunt

22. Romerica

"Romerica had a sinister plan....to corrupt its core values. Making men weak and scared of their own shadows. Producing fake facts, to drive into your living room, confusing you and even the pets too."

"Economic disasters, and open border mess, they soon found out, that it's never about. Tyrannical leaders, who keep their citizens divided. It may fall again, because of a fractured system. If we keep pushing this broken Romerica-last agenda."

"It's time to rise and start another day. You must open your eyes to finally see. America is a country that its citizens love and respect."

Join me in November, for we must end this shipwreck. Romeria will never fall. As we will share a victory lap. Trump as our president, finally America will be back."

"Reasoning behind this Poem"

'Rome fell because of selfish leaders, an open border, endless spending, a weak military, and a crushing economy. Now...compare exactly what's happening in America now. Romerica was written because of how America is today, and how it can become likened to Rome tomorrow, if things don't change course for the better.'

Thanks...Coffee Drinkers.

23. Texas Border

"Freedom rings from the soil of this great state. Americans finally making a stand against the devil's floodgate and illegal Aliens."

"National Guard, normal civilians, Truckers from all over the country...we all want what's best, for our borders and this great civilized nation. Safety and Security should be what we agree on...glad I don't live in a blue state...where the constitution doesn't belong."

"Biden needs illegals to roam free on this land, Texas had other plans. 25 states said we've had enough, sending American soldiers to stand united and finally being tough. A show of force...not seen since the last Civil War. Breaking ranks against the deep state. It's time to make this country great."

"The Texas Border is our last stand...we should unite...Afterall we are Americans. Some who gave it all to keep us free...from this textbook anti-Liberty Government Administration."

20. Brainwashed

"Progressed indoctrination, overreacting situations, overwhelming brainless functions. Mass incarceration, overseeding mindless thoughts. We are perfectly right...they are always wrong; it is where I belong. With my nonworking projective views, listening to the Mainstream media news."

"Forecasted beliefs, misinformed truths are what I see. It cannot be...tell me this is what I believe. Trump is bad, even though I cannot find. Anything other than outspoken disinformed Rymes. Telling me, the other 81 million are so blind."

"We are united with our government. They know what is best, finally got that off my chest. People just do not like it that we are going to win. Knowing we are never right; I can say that with a grin."

"Biden is good, as we are told...even though he is to dang old. So much for being brainwashed, as they all say. Time to put away my Paper Mache."

21. America Wins

"November 2024, we must unite and seek to elect. A man who can fix this broken system we all live in. We had it all, freedom, security, and a fine border wall. Cheap gas, diesel, and bread. Even the dogs & cats were fed."

"We must bring peace to the world, before we end up broke and alone. In America, that's being built for those corrupted divisive clones. People who bend laws to make it ok to target moms and dads for protesting love for the flag."

"Do what you must on election day...if you just get out and vote. For the person who will bring...an end to the deep state, finally cleaning government long-withstanding corrupted plates."

"This country will finally win...Let's all stick with Trump's master plan...To Make America Great Again...the end."

"Biden's America has me sinking. I cannot afford much to eat, so long to those dark and yummy treats. Burnt to a crisp just as I used to eat them. Replaced with dangerous chemicals, so much for that cookout this weekend."

"Red meat is something of the past, too bad it didn't last. For 30 + years, I never thought it would come to an end like that. Trying to save from Biden's divisive, brutal plan. To force us into eating crickets. I will go hungry, do you understand. Nothing good can come from man eating bugs for some sinister Globalist plan"

"Ramon Noodle soups 4 for a $1, can't pass that up, for saving a dollar. We must pay bills, to make ends meet, to work for nothing, living in a country who hates to provide. America is not supposed to starve its Citizens...sure wish Trump was back...instead of this wreck less, evil pride?"

"Guess what I am having for dinner tonight...My new dark and tasty treat. I have plenty to go around, stay a while, have a sit...come on in, grab a plate...don't be late, let's set a date, Ramon Noodles it is...Yummy...let us dig in."

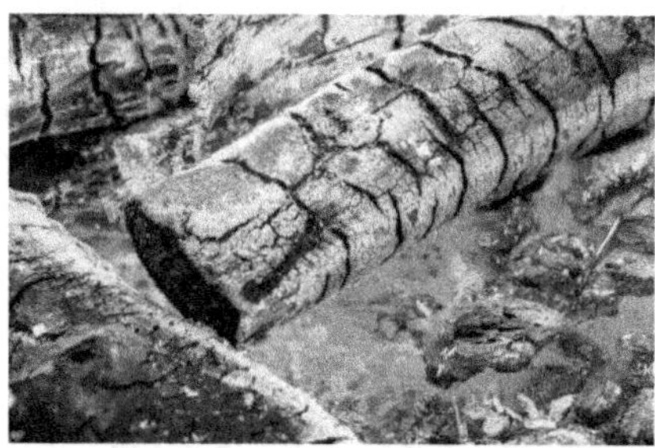

19. Satan's Army

"Careless trained actors, overreacting voids in our minds, dictating functional abilities, malfunctions...forced instability overloading our brains."

"Project Pride, Extremism, MK-Ultra, overthinking evaluations, psyops, false flags, shadowing the devil's delights. On the brink of war within ourselves...Nothing is off the table with their sinister news media fans."

"Blowing up fake vaccines, mandates, your rights vanishing, making you rethink your own self-worth...Putting you 4 feet underground, living in a fake reality, instructing your own demise in secret, bringing in the New World Order...just as planned."

"Controlling all narratives', Satan loves this division, as you try to overcome. The indoctrination of his plan...to seclude your birth rite from Lucifers army of fallen angels spread across this wasteland."

"We once called America...It's time to do grown up things, stop procrastinating, use your voice, never back down, Satan cannot win. After all God owns your soul...The End."

"X is a platform, where even dictators roam. Conservative values do not belong. Talking in a padded, forgotten room. Somewhere in the valley of misinformed views."

"Only those who pay will ever see their fate. For X is nothing more than a Globalists secret date. For substances of disinformed beliefs, do not be late...if you disagree...it is called hate."

"Extremism is real...but not as you are told. My opinions as an American should not be condemned, only to those who cannot see their own false reality they are living in.'

"X is owned by WEF, if you do not know this by now...you are just another liberal in the crowd. Who dictates what I can say, because of my faith, and making this country great."

17. The Meek & The Proud

"Doing everything on their own, asking for nothing in return. We seek to find another way out. For those who disbelief, or trust in our faith. Nothing is off the table for the meek who honors the father. We shall never falter."

"The proud find faults in others, but never look in their own mirrors. Judgement, stares, glares from the other side, of those rusted railroad tracks you live your stale-broken lives...sinking in debt, without an exit plan. People see others, only for self-gain, agree with me or you are out in the rain."

"Been there...done that, even with family. Your worth is so much more than those who don't share. Your accomplishments or praise the great job you have done. Nothing is good, unless you belong.'

"The Meek will inherit the earth, while the proud crumble in the quicksand of their own lust for your land. Without justifying anything... disagreeing with your life or trying to lead you astray."

The Meek Give...

"To those in need, because we are not proud, we come from the light, where peace and love exists. Not because we do not agree...but because of God's son, who died for our sins, so we could reap what we have sown...to keep our own bought and paid for home."

"The Meek will never be Proud...I hope you now understand...We are bound for the promise land."

18. Biden's 'Ramon Noodle Soup' America

"Nothing this life has to offer can overcome the division without the father, stepping to plate, never backing down, not stopping until we are united. He can heal all wounds, bow your heads let's get this great awakening started."

Prayer...

"Dear heavenly father, this world needs your help, we seek to find another path forward, without insights to our own struggles. Relating to justice in this free and Barron land, we give our lives to your master plan. You know what is right, what we are doing wrong, we cannot go on. Seeing each other in our divisive, anti-social minds."

"Please be with us, each day, while we battle Satan and his minions who deceive. Being proud, lusting over riches and fame, no one can hide from the devil's demise."

"Without you lord, this world is only going to get worse, separation, division, and distrust...even in government buildings, nothing is off the table. Satan has his grips, can't lose hope now, we must pray for this country, while we still can, let us all join in."

"Believe there is hope. For a better world, beyond the gates of evilness and hate. Nothing we do will ever be enough, for those who sacrifice us for their own greed they must."

"Your voice matters, it might look bad now...but Satan cannot win. He is Afterall...made from sin. Reach for the father, when you find no one to call, he can help your heart, heal from broken old wounds."

"Your past doesn't define who you can be. The future is bright, even for me. A sinner who can't cope with this broken reality, poverty-stricken, alone seeking to find. A world filled with love, understanding and value. Jesus said in the Bible...his children will never go through what they cannot handle."

A Divided World...

"Only for now...until Jesus steps in an and cleans up our sins, making us all whole again. We must keep fighting for a brighter, loving tomorrow. We will only get stronger...in faith & love for our father."

16. X

"Political voids shadowing this space. Division and hate because of our race. Elon bought Twitter and renamed it X. Powerful and united; freedom was at hand. Politicians who lie, cheat, and steal, tried to bring down this powerful man."

"Nothing we said would change our fate. Billionaires lust for what's beyond that gate. Freedom of Speech without Reach is nothing short of Censorship for those who teach. Silence is good, only if it is true. Conspiracies are the new facts they hide from you."

"Protests are a part of this country's strengths. Never underestimate those who diminish our rights. Taking your life...ask Ashlie how that one went, protesting for freedom, gets shot by a Policeman. He was never charged, but praised by others, never questioning his actions, even though she was unarmed. Ashie loved this nation, just wanted to protest a questioned election. Police let her in for her life to end."

"Arrested for supporting a person who made America great. Because if an election was not stolen, why make this their plan...Just trying to understand. Granma's went to jail for walking through a Capital, but Floyd rioters burnt police stations down and were let out of jail."

"Nothing is more sickening than seeing our nation struggling for answers. Justice for all, unless you voted for Trump. EPPS instructed and coerced you to move ahead...never arrested...must have been a FED."

"Our speaker was supposed to release the tapes, that proved it was set up to take our freedom away. Entrapment and silence from the left, more propaganda to prove. You are the problem...not the corrupted system in charge of the news."

"J6 was a history-making event. When government took down a president and his MAGA supporters. One day they will come clean, but not before the damage has been done. Political arrests and convictions for all who oppose. For a Police-State in the making, bringing down our Republic...I suppose."

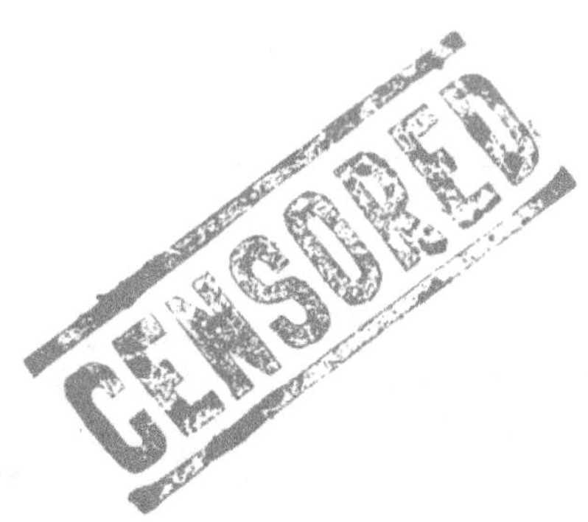

15. This Divided World.

"Division, Separation, institutional, irrationalism, People can't see to breathe can't believe what they hear the problems this world has. Even family can't feel your pain, the struggle to see the hate, I bet you can relate."

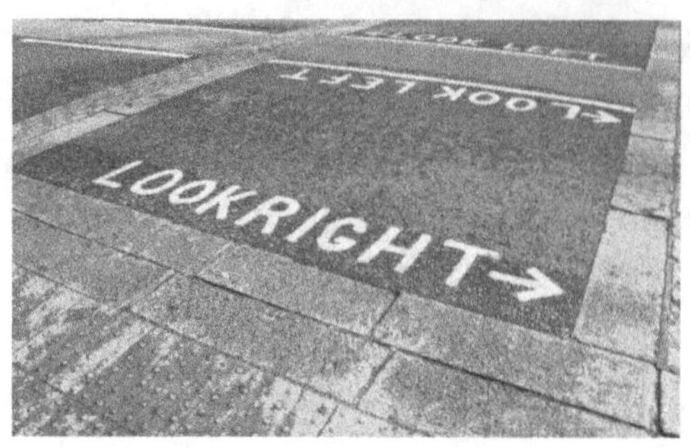

13. Border Walls

"Borders are for protection, from those who want what's yours. Jumping over the fence...wanting free rent. Illegals broke the law, but you are to blame. For not understanding, they are a sad and lonely diverse crowd."

"Chinese, Iranian, even Ukrainians too. They just want freedom like we all do. Military-aged men, plotting in secret to take over our land."

"Legal they are not...who really cares, 20 million plus, living among us now. Our President needs voters for another election to take down. They are walking around, destroying our cities and towns."

"Trump will end this chaos on day 1...rounding each up, sending them all home, where they belong. Come here legally, learn some history. Freedom is not free, and our borders cannot be open, to others who stomp on our constitution."

"Congress could have stopped this long ago but they ride the fence without using common sense. Posting on X, so we can have false hope. America can never be great, unless the border is secure, no walls, no justice for all."

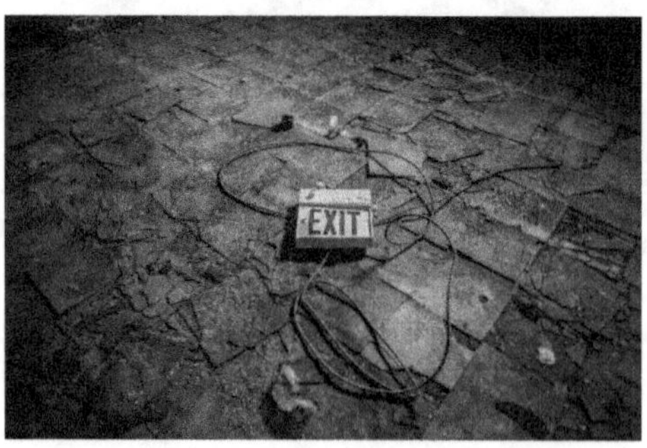

14. January 6th, 2021

Repent now before it is too late, no need to beg, just finish your plate. Before the Devil takes your soul away."

"Revivals in ever town and city we must do, seeking Jesus above the Devil's powerful few. Percentage of people longing for power, to feed your minds by indoctrinating design."

"Starting in schools, reaching the young, teaching boys they are young girls. Taking medications for the rest of their life. This was Afterall...The Devil's delight."

"The Bible says this is not the way, only those who deceive tell you to believe. God loves you no matter what, live as you please, don't read...God's word where it says. You must choose right from wrong... pray every day/night...he is watching from his heavenly home. Up there...in the sky."

12. Liberal Brainwashing

"Brainwashing is real, look over there, sheep in the field. Lost without a master, roaming around in circles, depending on government, waiting for enlistment. In a war they clapped on, a society they made themselves, time to pay up...welcome to the draft."

"Believing anything they see or hear, no time to check for facts, that would take up slack. In their endless broken chain, dragging on the ground, clowns flooding the streets, feeling a bit beat. Liberals know not what they do...they cry because they do not have a clue."

Except...

"The media and government are their programming channels, do not be late, under no circumstances. Trump is bad, Biden is good, even though you are poorer and miserable. Jobless, broke and without a home. 3 years in, it is all Trump's fault...let us just move on. Illegals roaming your streets, which is a good thing. Just give them your home...where it belongs."

"Brainwashing is something bad for most...but embracing this is something you must. Brainless Sheeple, repeating a mental forced disability. Liberals live in a washed-up false reality, banking on your ability to praise their own lustful adventures. Thoughtless choices, underestimating their mistakes."

"Society built this sinking ship...it is your right to learn something new. Never just believe the latest breaking news. Propaganda articles, and many false profits. We must pray for a better way. To learn and achieve greatness and gain power. From those who keep us down, for their own selfish greed."

10. Embracing Their Insanity

"Hatching out their plan, lusting for power, they misunderstand, we are living in a forgotten promise land, seeing all that's happening…still don't understand?"

"America was built for you and me, to see our full potential, while we stare into the sky. Waiting for Jesus to save us from those who are trying to break us. Can't you see, it is not for us to find. Only the upper class, for their own personal finance."

"With the tiny % of evil ones who are embracing their true insanity, building something for Illegals to make you a simple minority. Unless you wake up from your nightmarish false journey…nothing will be left if they continue to bow to Satan himself. Let them sink in their own swamp-filled quicksand. The Devil will never defeat Jesus in the end."

"Overreaching and arresting Americans by the thousands. Prebuilt concentration camps Gates put up his self. They are in a panic now. While you are Struggling to breathe underneath their dead/rotten trees."

"We must keep moving on, all warriors on social media, not backing down. Information warfare, critical thinking, question everything, never just trust. The sky is clearing up, you and I will never give up…The clouds will be gone soon enough…When Trump makes America…Great…Again…Amen."

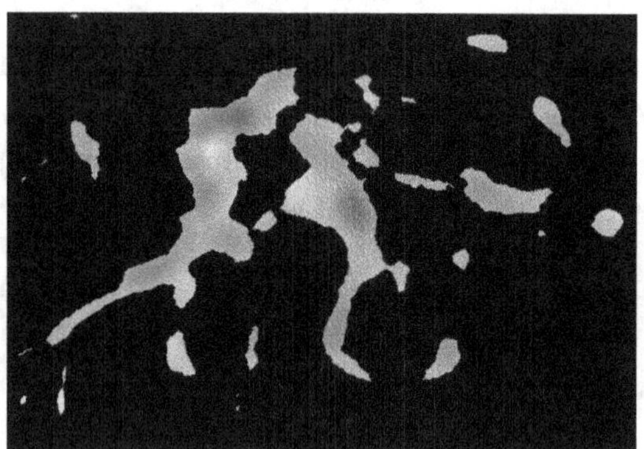

11. Live as You Please

"They have fallen from grace, our country is in decline, many are lost in their prideful-sinful lusts. Sacrificing the majority, for an evil delight. In Satan's hand, this land has gone…betrayed God and America's golden plan."

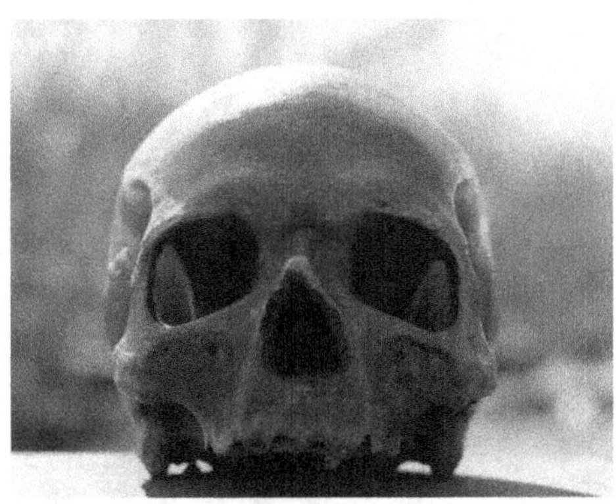

9. Elephants are Red, Donkeys are Blue

"Elephants are Red, Donkeys are Blue, this country's colors are not for you to construe. Not a Democracy, it's led by a constitution. Too bad the Donkey's don't own this institution."

"Elephants are strong, while Donkey's are weak and frail, it shows on a wide-open scale. Power corrupts their minds, causing them to go blind."

"Elephants get arrested For Political gain by those who are so blue, like China and Iran, a Police State we live, what country do we really have left."

"Projective Extremists united the Donkey's stand until their ship ran upon the sand. Next November, it is time to vote again. It will not be like you are told. Trump will win and Make America Great. That was always his plan."

"Lies being told, because Donkey's can't think on their own. Sheep have no self-control. Until they finally let go. Of the brainwashed ideals, their masters instill in their souls."

"Elephants and Donkeys have nothing in common. We love America, the others control the narrative."

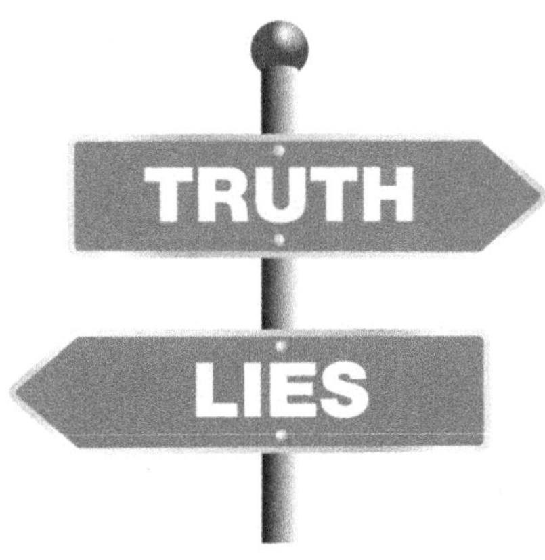

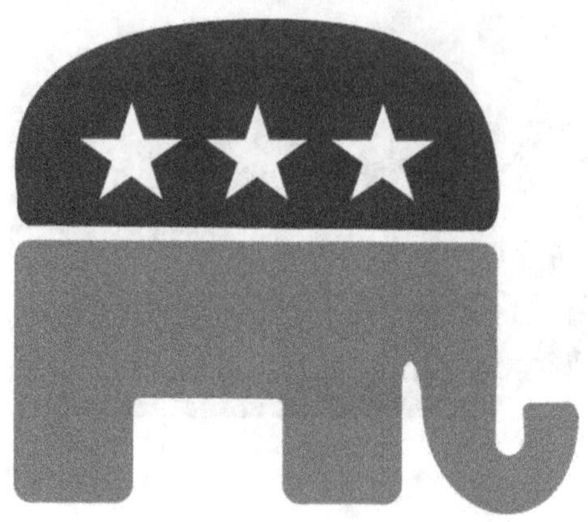

8. The Devil is Back

"He never gives up, destroying everything he touches in sight. One false move, Satan will take over a Country. Pride on the streets, even in our government offices. Nothing beats the Devil, with God pushed out into the forbidden shadows."

"Once a great nation, America stood strong. Now it is all gone...with the Devil sitting on his worldly throne. This planet is being swept in the trash with an evil-barbaric broom. With Lucifer lurking around in every classroom."

"The lies are told daily, from every sad, depressing angle. The media, and government agencies, working together against God's creation."

"The world is at war; can't say you were not told. Satan rose up inside of these corrupted wealthy-worldly agents. Bringing division once again to this peaceful loving Planet"

"They string up your rights, preventing your freedoms. Shaking down the Christian religion. In the name of justice for all, but not for you. Preventing you to preach but allowing terror-related riots in the streets."

"We are living in a corrupted political equation. Prayer can bring us back from this pending disaster. Putting God back...where he belongs...in power."

"I'm just saying what you all are thinking, can't stop now, running out of gas, coasting downhill, nowhere to go, because of the out-of-control freakshow. Who Cators to the 1%, forcing 99% to comply or be condemned. Social Media, MSM, or Radio it's all the same Lying propaganda news."

"Thanks to Bidenomics, the poor are now poorer, the middle class is now broken, and the rich can buy your homes you are foreclosing on soon.

More government programs, and free shit for illegals. While homeless Americans get absolutely f$&king nothing. But a few government-supplied drugs to pass around to the crowd.

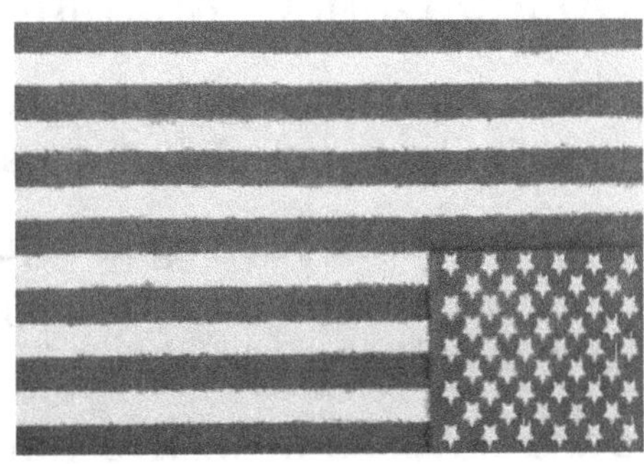

7. Game Over 2024

"When the game is finally over, and WEF is batting zero. When the Deep State is no more, and the Clowns are crying, rolling on the floor."

"Will America finally be free from the people who disbelieved. In the Making America Great Again, it was Afterall God's master plan...don't you see."

"Trump will win again, even though Democrats will try to install. Another batshit crazy to take the fall."

"For all Obama's dirty laundry Michelle must upkeep and store. For his big break to win, trying to sing that division song once again."

"Hidden around closed doors, in the subbasement below. Where evil lurks beneath the creaking steps. Biden's basement Liberals wait."

"For the time to come out screaming like all liberals do, for the judgement is at hand. Trump won in 2024...You're fired...this is the end."

"MAGA is a threat to democracy, loving America is dangerous too. Spoken by a true tyrannical governing extremist, who hates this country 1000% times more than you do."

"Loving God is a sin while pride is flooding across this land. Hate, Violence is praised as protests, better not hide your face."

Love and Diversity...means Division, governing by race, indoctrinating your children, according to the Deep State."

"Democratic Projection we see every single day. Corrupt officials, bending your mind, causing most to go blind."

5. The Coffee Drinker Morning Show

"Welcome coffee drinkers, to this fantastic show. It is filled with people from all over the globe. Time to research, find the truth, unlike all the mainstream media news."

"Fearless Americans, standing up to tyrants, pushing an agenda for the tiny percentage. Question everything you see, because you're living around a bunch of brainless/braindead sheep."

"Bring out your coffee mugs and stay for a while. Every morning before the break of dawn. The Coffee Drinker Morning Show will be on."

"The time is now when we must unite. It won't be long before this world will be gone. Because of corrupted people running the country. It's now or never...so I've been told. Hold on to your hats...it's time to go"

"Every single day...Monday through even Sunday. Welcome everyone...let's try to get along. We're not like those liberals who cry/complain all day long...."

6. BIDENOMICS

"Broke and in despair, lost in this world. Seeking food from the public pantry, hoping to not lose my sanity. Bidenomics has me starving for something better. Maybe I'll just write a letter."

Letter Says...

"No money, losing time as we speak, shit health, poverty striction, lost my wealth to greedy f&%king government politicians."

Bidenomics hit my home like a train running full speed. Lost everything I own, now I'm broke and all alone. Could you spare some rice, maybe a couple bricks of government bread...not too picky, living in this strange foreign land."

"People think our flag is just a piece of cloth. They Just don't understand what it really cost. Men and Women, who fought and died, to keep our flag from falling on the ground. Off the deserts of countries far and wide. Friends, brothers, sisters, fathers, and mothers, who died to keep it flying in the sky."

"The Flag flies for those who gave their life, sacrificed with blood/sweat/tears, to give you a right to disrespect those colors while sitting on your ass."

"To keep you from being the family who gets a knock on their door. At 3am, telling you your family member when to heaven for fighting to keep that flag off the floor."

"You may just soon find out what our flag's all about. The draft will prove to you...the flag's colors are more than just...red, white, and blue. For a reason, you might not have learned. From your Social Media platform."

-American Flag Color Meaning-

"Valor and Bravery for those who taught our enemies a lesson. About the Purity and Innocence of our flag, showing them Vigilance, Perserverance, and justice for all. Because America never backs down...from tyrants disrespecting the Red, White, and Blue."

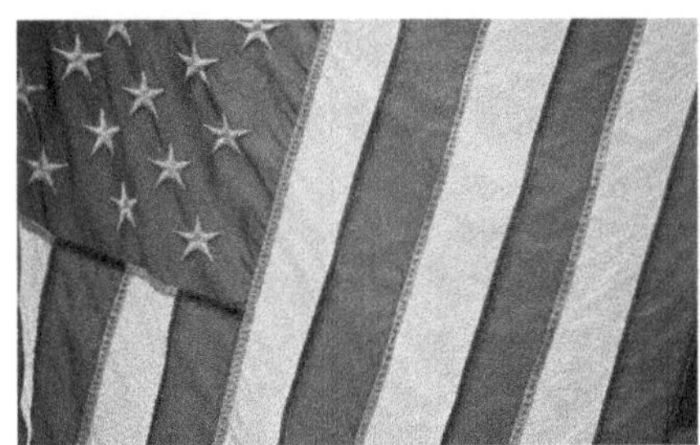

4. Democratic Projection

"Democratic Projection sharing their real views, spreading lies, and disowning the truth. Sacrificing our freedom, for their own guilty pleasures. The Devil owns their souls, above and beyond all measures."

"Democratic Projection represented by the media. Truths are conspiracies in the shadows of misinformed opinions. Thoughtless ideals, bankrupting America. Funding every country but our own damn nation."

2. Trump 2024

"40-Year inflation, 23-Year High FED rates too, there must be some big mistake, or We're just as blind as Liberals too. Endless government spending, I sure don't feel very Rich. We are worse off than Biden's depends after a chocolate ice cream glitch."

"91 Felony charges, 2 impeachments, and a few investigations later. Trump got arrested for something Democrats done better."

"The FBI and DOJ. Are they not supposed to be good guys/gals? Why are they being used by the Deep State now, to put Trump away, so we will never see. The real corrupt works of Hunter & Joe's art galleries."

"Because secrets hold their value, if you're very rich. Nothing can break the chains from those black books kept in Clinton's secret digital vault. By the gatekeeper of these powerful government agents. Who disregarded our constitution, because they must prevent their Demons. From ever coming to conclusion."

Trump 2024...

"Trump made America great, even for those who hated his Tweets. He drove peace into the world, never thinking about himself. Lies have been told, the damage been done."

"America is strong, because its people understand. 2024 is the last stand. Trump will clean the corrupt people once and for all...from this wonderful, amazing land...the end."

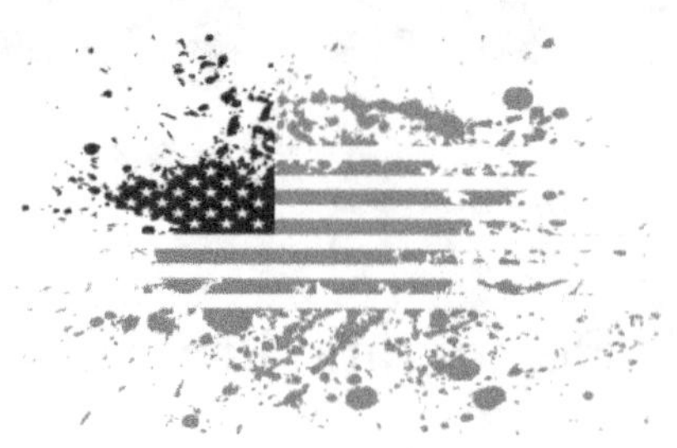

3. American Flag

(Dedicated to my brother)

(Army Special Forces 20 years).

1. Ukraine's Money

"$1 billion, $20 billion, $100 billion...who cares at this point. It's all Fake money, spent by crooks. Taxed to the ends of this earth, even after death. The government says it is money well spent."

"Helping a Democracy, who is not even in NATO, corrupt to its core...just ask Joe. Obama/Biden spent time away, in 2014, it all went wrong. Snipers on rooftops, shooting all who stood against. Ukraine was free at last...Says the corrupted left."

"No one questioned anything. Because we enjoy the view. From our living rooms, watching the tube. The Ukrainian government was overthrown, not long afterwards, their citizens came back home."

"Silent backroom meetings, most are unknown. Hold out your hands, time to pay up. Says the 85,000 new IRS agents, knocking on your doors."

"The Media says Ukraine is at war, but no news crews on the ground. Zelensky's wife has offshore accounts, with money free flowing in every town."

"Taxpayer-funded Ukrainian vacations, there is no accountability where the money's gone. Politicians love to preach the same boring song. Support Ukraine, keep sending your taxes. Listen to us, we know what is best. We are from the Government and we're your friends"

'The Coffee Drinker'

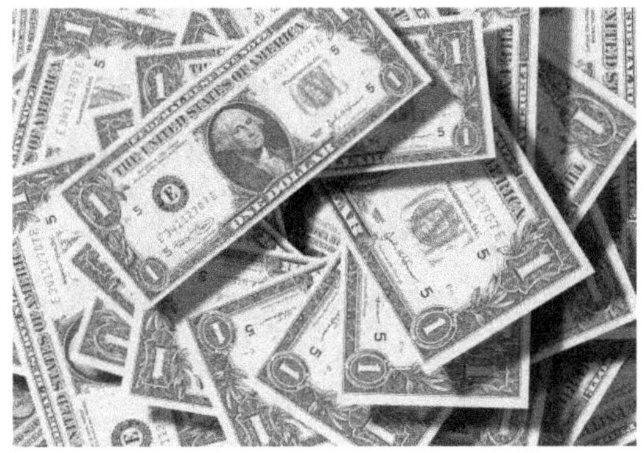

PROLOGUE:

‘The Thought Process Behind these 25 Political Poems’

The last 3 + years have opened my mind to what America is having to endure. Chaos on our southern border, endless spending by Politicians, and wars and rumors of wars.

These poems were written and shared on my social media page upon completion. You now have in your hands poems that show exactly what you have been going through. How crazy the last couple of years have been, and how much we need stability back in the White House.

Taxpayer-funded money laundering in Ukraine, to forced objective inclusion in wars overseas. An invasion at our southern border, to uncontrolled drugs pouring in from China.

Poetry gives us something to read, while the world crumbles around our feet. It shows the average side of life. The life of someone who buys their own groceries, pays for their own gas, and works to make ends meet. In a failing country that’s been through it all.

I hope you enjoy these poems, as it was a joy to write them for you.

Thank you for being here...Coffee Drinkers.

‘The Coffee Drinker’